WOMEN'S TRAINING GUIDE TO SEXY FIT ARMS

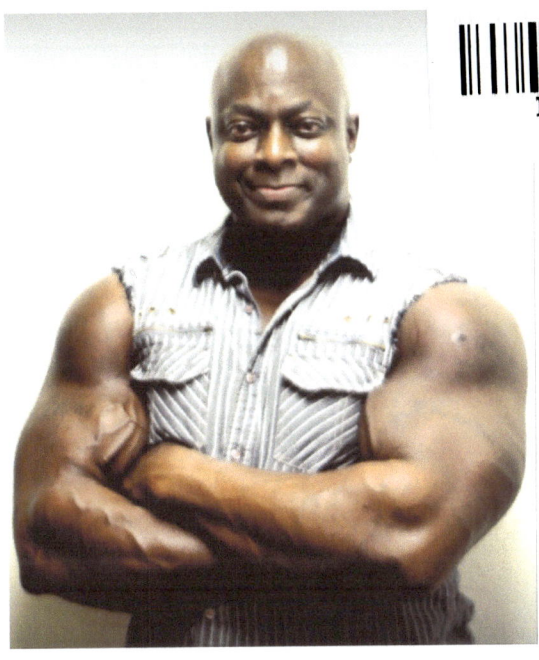

I0435779

Copyright © 2016 by Daryl Jones

Women's Training Guide To Sexy Fit Arms
By Daryl BIG"D" Jones

Table of Contents

Women's Training Guide To Sexy Fit Arms
By Daryl BIG"D" Jones

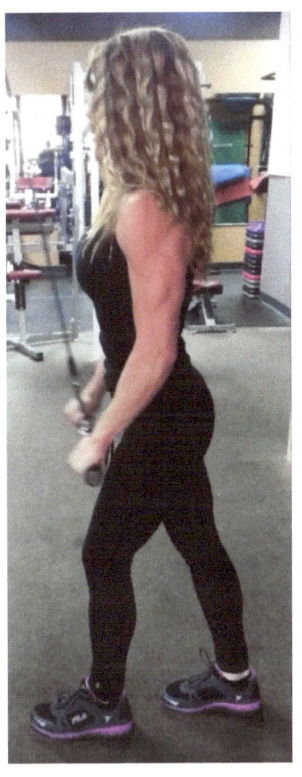

Women's Training Guide To Sexy Fit Arms is intended to be used for general guidelines only and no exercise of any kind, including those in this book, should be attempted without first consulting with a doctor and determining your physical suitability for strenuous exercise. The results in the book are not guaranteed and individual results will vary depending on many factors not addressed in this book.

Foreword

My name is Daryl Jones I was born an only child in Berkeley, California, and raised by my single mom in Los Angeles. My mom worked hard to raise me as best she could and looking back I must say she did an awesome job as I wanted for nothing due to her many, many sacrifices in life for me (thanks mom). Growing up in Los Angeles was tough, so in 1974 my mom decided to pack us up and move to the great northwest Portland Oregon.

I hated the move as I was at the ripe age of 9yrs old I had no say in the matter at all. Looking back I realize like most parents mother knew best, as we lived in an area that was much less busy compared to where we lived in Los Angeles. Though at the age of nine I didn't really understand why my mom did what she did. Looking back I realized that not only did she take me to a much safer environment, she also basically saved my life as I'm sure that I would have become a complete product of my environment.

Women's Training Guide To Sexy Fit Arms
By Daryl BIG"D" Jones

Being in Portland also gave a few different male role models to follow in my family and the main one was my grandfather (Papa JJ) he was a man of all men, tough when he needed to be and always very kind, but what made me see him differently than all the rest was his endless love for his family. My grandfather was also a man of dignity and a man with deep family values. He instilled in me just how important it was to work hard at all that you do. My grandfather got up at the same time every morning, work or no work you could set your clock to the squelching sound of the shower coming on at 3am every single day of the week. This is why I say today that nothing comes to a sleeper but a dream, and in order for that dream to become a reality you have to get up and work towards that dream on a daily basis in order for it to become a reality. This leadership example that he and my uncles set before me has made me who I am today and I'm very thankful for that upbringing.

-Daryl BIG"D" Jones

1. Introduction

Most men don't believe that women can accomplish the same fitness goals as they do. The truth is quite the opposite, in fact not only can women accomplish the same fitness goals, but the truth be told women (in my opinion) have a higher level of discipline, than "most" men. Now the reason I say these things are from my own personal observation over the past 36 years in the gyms across the country. Now about the only thing that women in the fitness world can't do the same as men is grow equally as large as a man.

For men or anyone else to think or believe that women can't accomplish similar goals such as developing their arms to become not only well defined and toned but also having the ability to increase the strength of their arms, is not only wrong but is also displaying a very shallow style of thinking. Now in the old days it was very common to believe that women can't do as men do in many areas of life, but as time has gone by this way of thinking has been proven to be incorrect.

Women's Training Guide To Sexy Fit Arms
By Daryl BIG"D" Jones

Women have not only proven this way of thinking to be wrong time and time again, but over the years women have been allowed to more freely participate in such events as simply going in to a gym and lifting weights as men do. We have since seen countless women do the once thought to be impossible and now proven to be possible and this includes having stronger muscles. Not only have women now been doing this for quite some time but they have also taken those proven capabilities to even higher levels.

Two women who are now known as the first "ever" women to become US Army Rangers, First Lt. Shaye Haver and Capt. Kristen Griest, on August 21st 2015 these two women accomplished the once thought to be physically as well as mentally impossible for any woman to ever successfully achieve, and that was to past a series of the most intense physically challenging test that the US armed forces has ever compiled to become a US Army Ranger. To fully understand the magnitude of this accomplishment, you'd have to understand that most men fail this goal during the first four days of RAP (Ranger Assessment Phase).

Women's Training Guide To Sexy Fit Arms
By Daryl BIG"D" Jones

Now I mention these two women as they are not only the most recent to make American history, but they made history by breaking down another thought to be impossible physical barrier created by men, placed on women as no woman has ever passed and graduated the US Army's Rangers training program. To become a US Army Ranger is one of the most physical challenges known to man and is known to be arguably the toughest training in the entire US Armed Forces. To understand just how incredible the feat that these two women have accomplished is, let's take a close look at the count-less amount men of all walks throughout the history of the mere existence of the Army Rangers, that have fallen short of completing this same exact physical accomplishment and let's not forget the mental strength that had to be involved here.

So to get back to my point discussed earlier, to believe that women in the fitness world can't or aren't capable of accomplishing the same (or similar) physical goals as men, is not only far from being true but a very primitive and incorrect way of thinking period. History has shown us once again that this an out dated way of thinking.

Women's Training Guide To Sexy Fit Arms
By Daryl BIG"D" Jones

So ladies if you desire your arms to become sexy and fit, let's start by focusing on just that, by saying I can and I will have the arms I so desire. This is all possible with my proper training technique along with proper nutrition.

Equal Opportunity

In the fitness world you can be Oprah Winfrey, Taylor Swift or just an ordinary every day woman, you only get out of training what you put into training. In the fitness world you don't have to have a college degree, nor a huge budget, heck let's be honest you don't even need to have a job to change the way your body looks. All you really need is what I call the 3D Principals, Dedication, Determination & Discipline. Heck, if you really think about it you don't even need weights to change the way you look. Push-ups and sit ups are 100% free and no one can stop you but you.

2. The 3D Principle

The 3D Principal stands for Dedication, Determination and Discipline, this is something I have followed nearly me entire life. I started using it with all my clients years ago in the belief of a person with these principals can accomplish not only their fitness goals but in most all goals they set in life "if" they truly stick to the 3D Principals. I'm a firm believer that when a person decides to make major changes in their life either in fitness or in other aspects, they can better achieve their set goals with the 3D principals.

I have used these three principals in my own fitness goals and have never been disappointed by my end results. By using the these principals I've always known that I've given it my all, 110% and knowing that alone has always made me feel like a winner at the end of the day. Let's discuss what these principals actually are and what they mean to me in the world of fitness.

Dedication

To never allow yourself to make any excuses that prevents you from working towards achieving your fitness goals on a daily basis. Some days you may or may "not" feel like training but here's where your dedication comes in and you train anyway. So many times in life we cross paths with people who use words like, I'm about to or I'm getting ready to, these words all sounds like excuses to not be dedicated. You have to be dedicated to achieve any goal you set in life no matter if it's developing sexy, fit arms or losing a few unwanted pounds.

Dedication has to be a part of your plan in order to successfully achieve your set goals. Don't be one of those people who is always "about" to do this or is "about" to do that, be a person who is dedicated to finish the goals you have set for yourself. You see being dedicated and working out isn't about the short term goals alone it's about the lifetime rewards of pushing yourself hard to create a healthier you that will definitely last a lifetime.

Women's Training Guide To Sexy Fit Arms
By Daryl BIG"D" Jones

So many of us think that training will only make us look better, when the fact is training on a regular basis will also aide us in preventing future illnesses, you can call this a sort of preventive medicine. It is so important to stay focused and dedicated to each realistic physical goal we set, whether it's developing a set of sexy fit arms or dropping a few unwanted pounds. Dedication is a key role player and without dedication you will surely fall short of your initial set goals.

Determination

To stay focused and finish the fitness goals you started and allowing nothing to make you ever quit or give up, shows a person's level of determination. Let's all face one fact and that is quitting is always the easy way out of accomplishing or fitness goals "but" when we're determined to and dedicated to our goals we are much more likely to succeed.

Women's Training Guide To Sexy Fit Arms
By Daryl BIG"D" Jones

You see determination is a mindset, so let's not allow our minds to place limits on what's so achievable by keeping ourselves focused to finish what we started. Setting limits on our minds will prevent us from achieving most of the goals that we've ever thought about going after. Determination will keep us so focused on what we've set our minds to accomplish that we'll be totally oblivious to anything attempting to distract us from our fitness goals. The power of determination will keep our focus on starting and actually finishing the goals we set for ourselves allowing nothing to stray us off our individual goals.

Determination requires a different type of mind set, it requires using more powerful words towards ourselves, such as I can, I must and I will. Determination is what is going to push us through the struggles that often occur during the training session, as well as keep us on track with our nutrition. Determination is what's going to help drive us towards, developing a sexy fit set of arms.

Discipline

Discipline is a must in order for us to bring this all together. You have to be disciplined to work toward you fitness goals on a daily basis. Discipline will never allow you to miss your training, or forget to eat your meals on time. Discipline will have you prepare you meals today for tomorrow and discipline will have you stay punctual on, going to the gym on time as well as going to bed on time and getting the much needed rest and for proper recovery.

Discipline plays such an important role in simply dealing with all that life throws at us and we all know life can and most likely will throw us a few curve balls from time to time that's just how life is, "but" with discipline you can not only get through those curve balls but you can stay focused and make the necessary adjustments to stay on track with the fitness goals that you have set for yourself.

Women's Training Guide To Sexy Fit Arms
By Daryl BIG"D" Jones

Discipline is such a powerful tool to have, discipline will take you to new journeys and new levels in life. Discipline is a must to have in order to achieve the goals you have set for yourself in life, in the gym and out. Discipline will be a huge contributor towards your success, discipline along with your intense determination and dedication will definitely make you stand out from the rest.

Dedication, determination along with discipline will help you achieve your fitness goals with the greatest of ease. You can see how all three of these seem to really say or point to the same direction, and if you truly apply these three principals you will find that in the end of your journey you came out with some pretty successful results in developing your very own set of sexy fit arms. So train hard and train consistently and use the 3D principals and you to will have your very own success story to tell.

MENTAL FOCUS (FIND IT AND FEEL IT)

I personally always tell my clients to find the muscle and feel it. What am I actually saying here? I'm saying to make that mind to muscle connection that we all have subconsciously. Let's take a moment and close our eyes, now make a fist and begin to move your arm up and down as though you were flexing your bicep. Now as you are moving your arm up and down really start to mentally focus on every fiber moving as your arm moves in this upward and downward motion.

This may seem or sound strange right now but as you are becoming more seasoned in your training you will find that by becoming more in tuned with your body you'll be taking your workouts to a totally different level and your training will "feel" explosive. On a lot of sets (not all) I'll close my eyes and get so deeply in tuned with the body part that I'm training, that I'm able to block out the normal level of that burning sensation that we all get, to where I'm able to push past that point giving myself the much needed ability to complete my entire set without the normal signs of fatigue.

Women's Training Guide To Sexy Fit Arms
By Daryl BIG"D" Jones

Now let's be clear on something here, I'm still feeling the burn the same as anyone else, but with this deep focus I'm able to minimize the burning and push past where most will simply stop. The other benefit of becoming in tuned with your muscles is that you'll be able to create more of what I call, hidden strength, opposed to the person who simply just walks up and grabs a barbell or dumbbell with no mind to muscle connection (no focus at all). Understand that for most this will take time to master and for some depending on your training background you'll discover this technique fairly quickly.

Unfortunately for some of you this connection may never be made, sorry but over the years I'm seen so many try but for whatever reason they just aren't able to make this mind to muscle connection. For those of you who are able to make this connection between your mind and your muscles, this connection will definitely up your game in the gym as well as up your game in your overall training performance. Just be willing to give it a try and be willing to also give it time, as all in this fitness world all things takes time as well as effort. Now go train and find the muscle and feel it.

3. Workout

Now let's train and start developing those sexy and fit arms.

Skull crushers
Standing barbell curls
Cable press downs (straight bar)
Dumbbell hammer curls
Body weight dips
Side laterals

TRICEPS (EXERCISE #1)
Skull Crushers

Now let's start training and let's begin with the all to famous skull crushers also known as kick-outs and let's load it with a fairly controllable weight using a straight bar. Make sure that you don't load this up with a over challenging weight as we will be doing 4 set of 25 repetitions for our triceps (the upper back part of the arm) with very little rest in between each set.

Women's Training Guide To Sexy Fit Arms
By Daryl BIG"D" Jones

The goal is to perform the first set of 25 repetitions and take a short rest of 60 seconds. Then immediately begin the second set of 25 repetitions and repeat the 60 seconds of rest. Then begin set number three and repeat until you have successfully completed all four sets of 25 repetitions, equaling a total of 100 repetitions.

Now the reality is that most of you will need to stop and rest in the middle of the set. This is normal until you get your body conditioned to a higher level and then you'll be able to conduct all four sets with stopping any longer than the 60 seconds specified in between each set. For those who do need to rest in the middle of the 25 repetition set, try not to rest for longer than 15-30 seconds and resume where you left off at in your count, until you reach 25 repetitions.

TRICEPS (EXERCISE #1)
**Skull Crushers 4 set's of 25 repetitions
100 repetitions total.**

Grip the bar with thumbs on top.

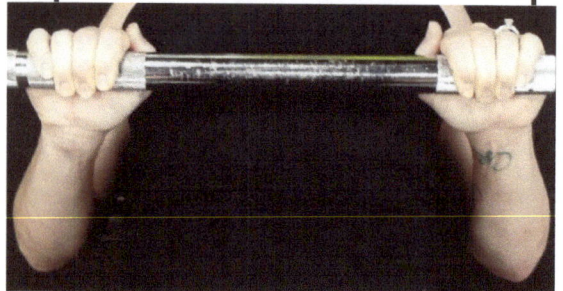

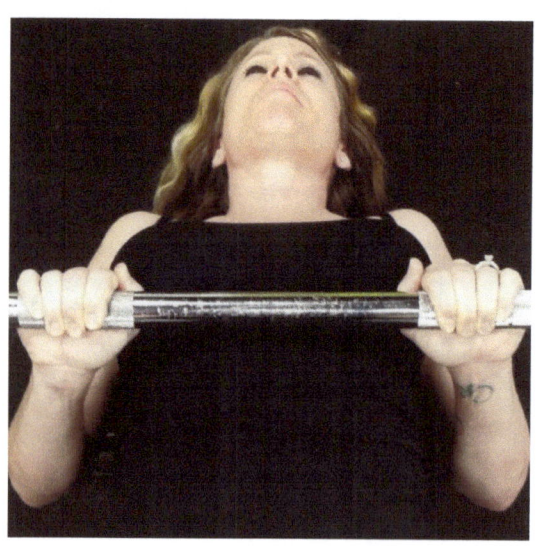

Rest on chest if or when needed.

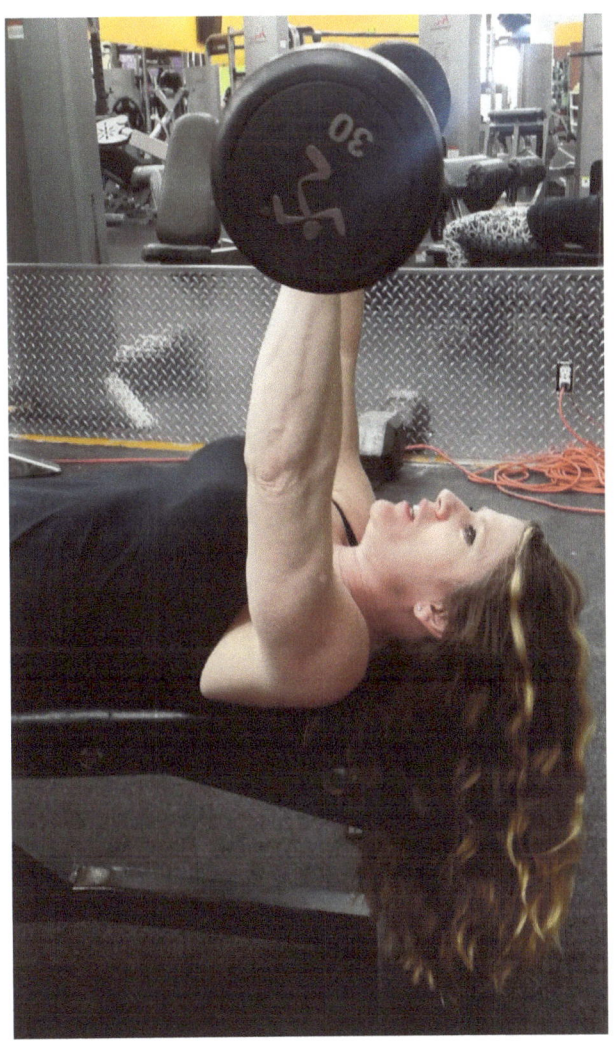

At the top of this movement, begin to inhale just before bringing the weight downward.

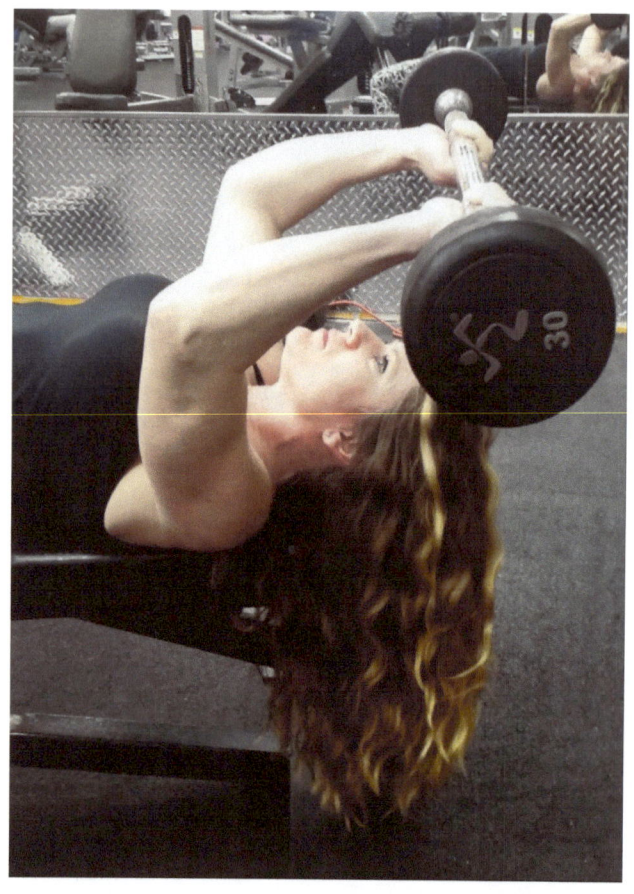

Continue inhaling as you're bringing the weight downward. Also keep a tight hand grip on the bar, as this will give you more power as you're performing this movement.

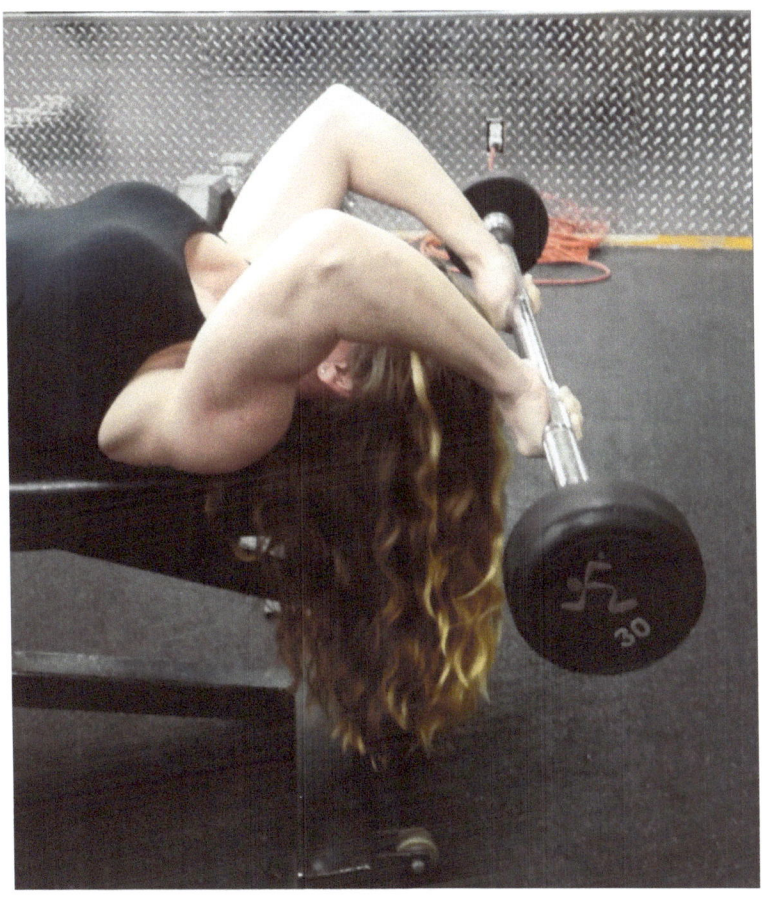

**Now just before powering the weight
upward begin to exhale, but don't fully
exhale until you are at the top/completion
of the repetition.**

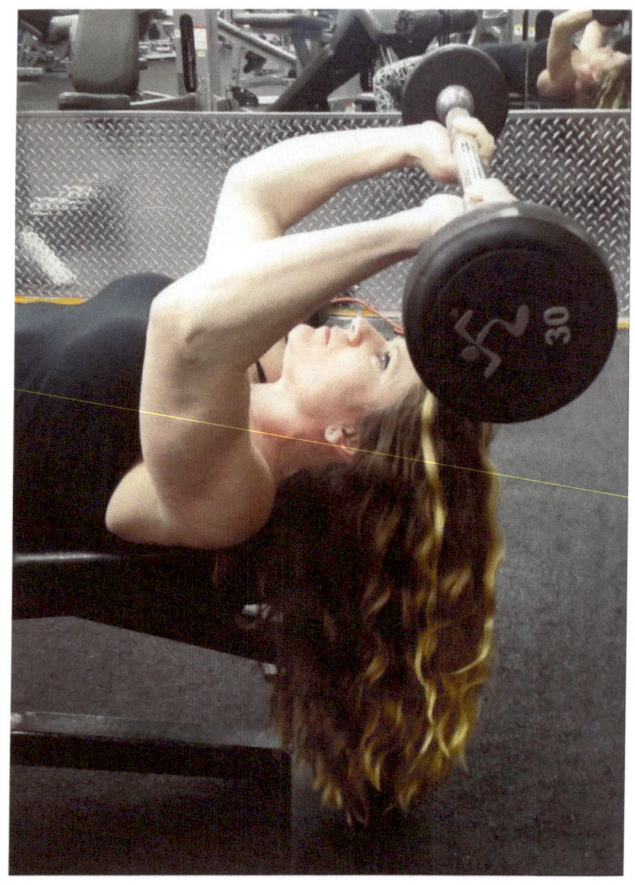

Continue to blow out (exhaling) as you are bringing the weight back upward.

Women's Training Guide To Sexy Fit Arms
By Daryl BIG"D" Jones

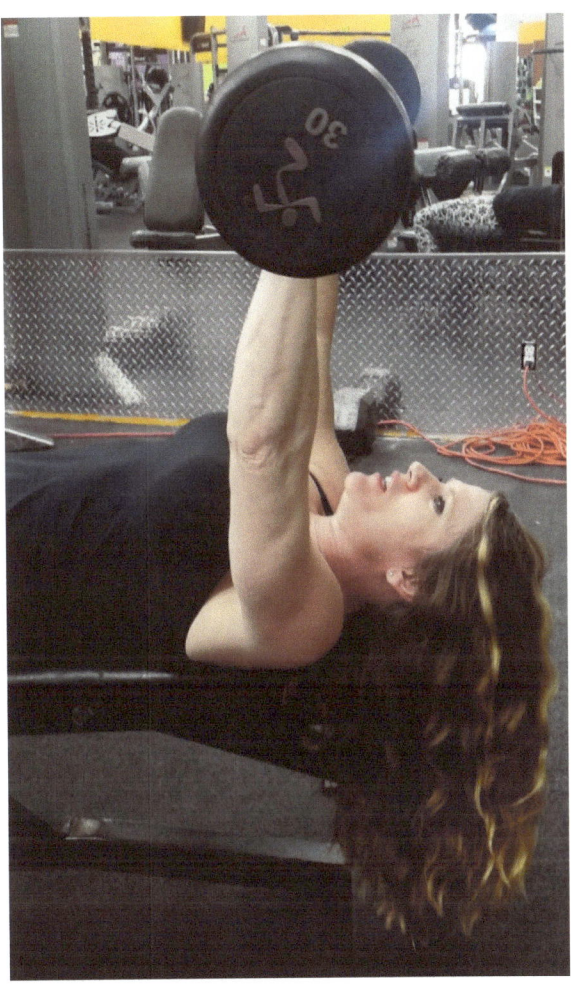

As you return to the top of this movement fully exhale and repeat for 25 reps for 4 sets, 100 reps in total. Remember to only rest for 60 seconds in between each set.

Standing Barbell Curls

Now that our triceps are full of blood with a good pump, let's now focus on our biceps with a traditional straight bar standing barbell curl, using a standard shoulder width grip. Select a weight that you know is light weight enough for you complete 25 repetitions straight for 4 sets, making your total count, 100 repetitions, just as we did above with the skull crushers.

Remember try your best not to rest for longer than 60 seconds between sets. This will be tough but you can do it. If you start to tire do as many as you can and split the reps if needed into repetitions of 5 for example if you are rep 10 and you decide you need to rest, don't set the weight down "but" take a breather and then make a 5 rep commitment and go for 15 reps and so on, until you complete the entire 25 repetitions. Ok we're not done with our training yet so let's get back to training.

Standard hand grip.

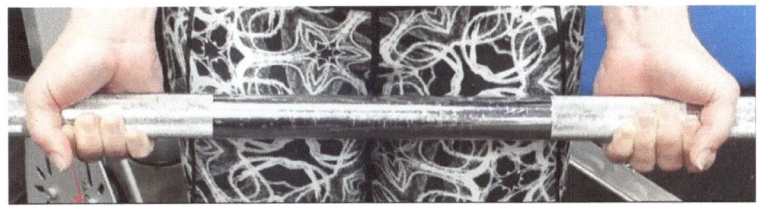

Here we'll use a traditional standard hand grip as we perform the standing barbell curl. By gripping the bar tightly you may find that you will discover additional strength to perform this exercise. We also will want to focus on correct breathing patterns, which will be explained in the photos below each illustrated photo. Breathing properly will definitely maximize your ability to complete each set of 25 repetitions, just as improper breathing will definitely hinder your full potential in performing this exercise.

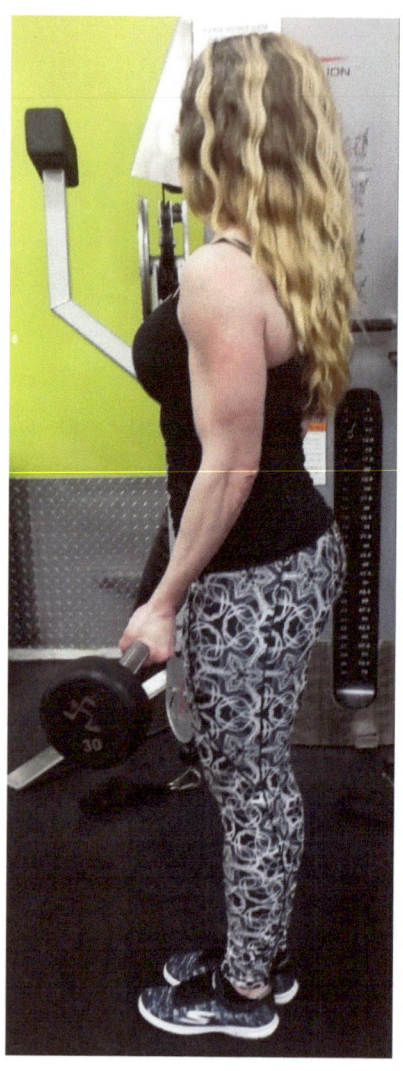

Take a deep breath, filling up your lungs and just before curling upward begin to exhale.

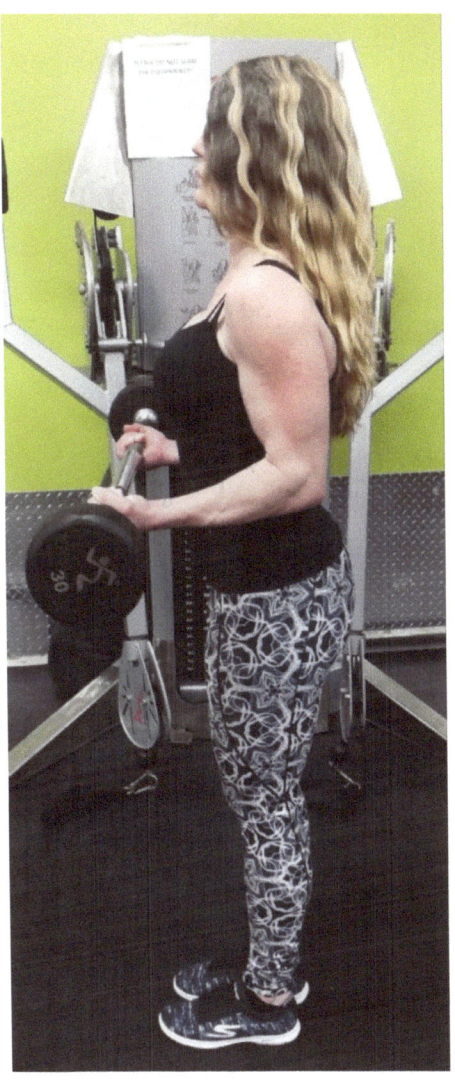

Continue to blow out (exhaling) as you are curling the weight upward.

Women's Training Guide To Sexy Fit Arms
By Daryl BIG"D" Jones

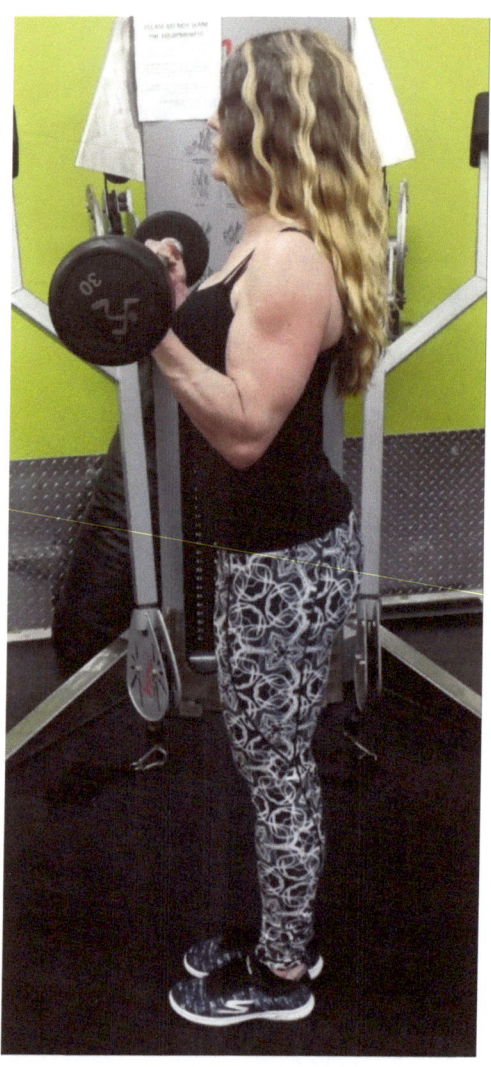

Now fully exhale at the top and repeat for 25 reps. Do 4 sets of 25reps for a total of 100 repetitions.

Cable Press Downs

Now let's return back to our triceps and let's now do another 4 sets of 25 repetitions with the exact same rest periods as above 60 second in between if training alone and if training with a workout partner rest only while your training partner is performing their set of 25 reps. By now I'm sure at this point you can see the importance of your mind being set for achievement as this is going to a game of mental strength as well as physical strength.

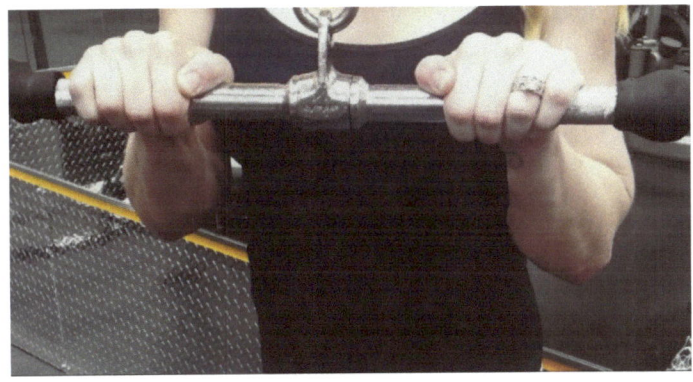

Thumbs on top.

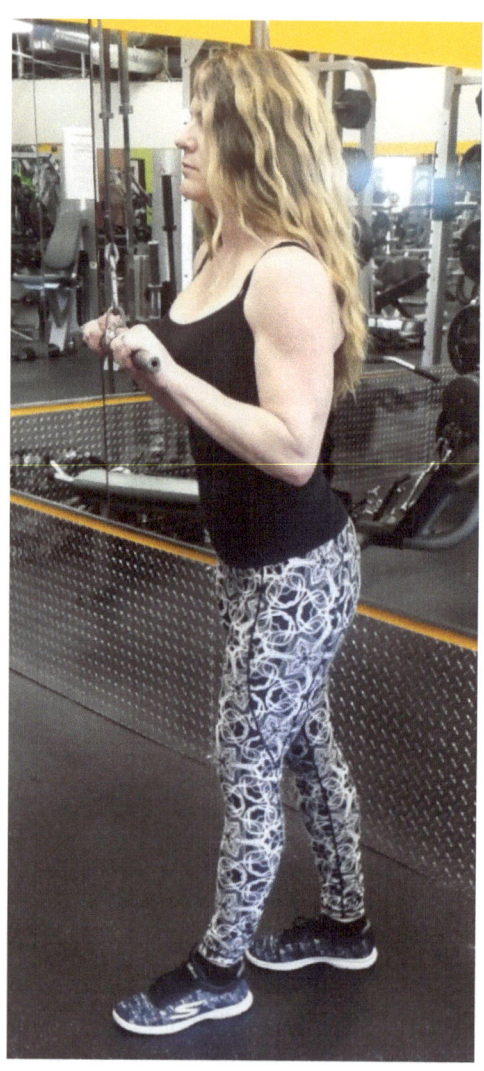

Lean slightly inward towards the cable, take a deep breath (side view) and just before pressing downward, begin to exhale.

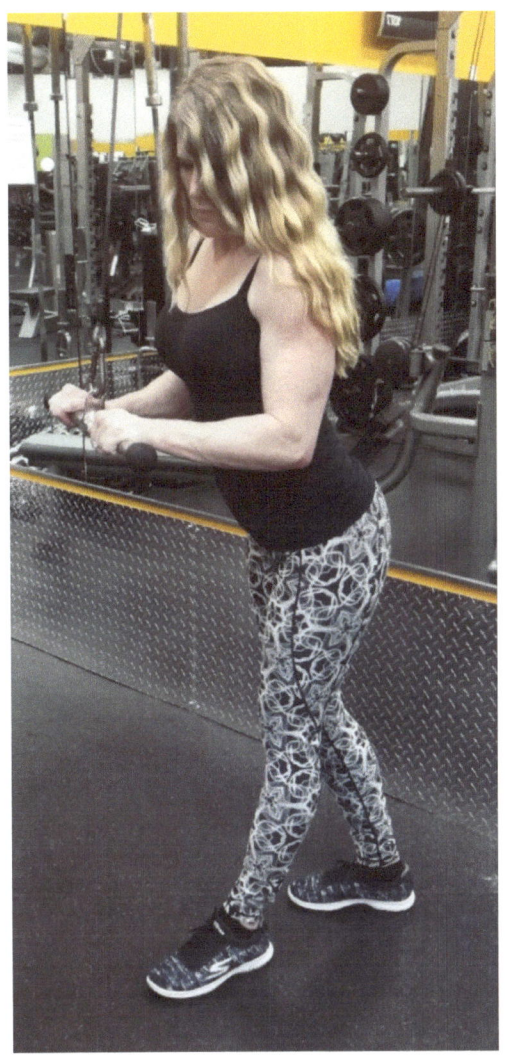

Continue exhaling (blowing out) as you're pressing the cable straight bar downward.

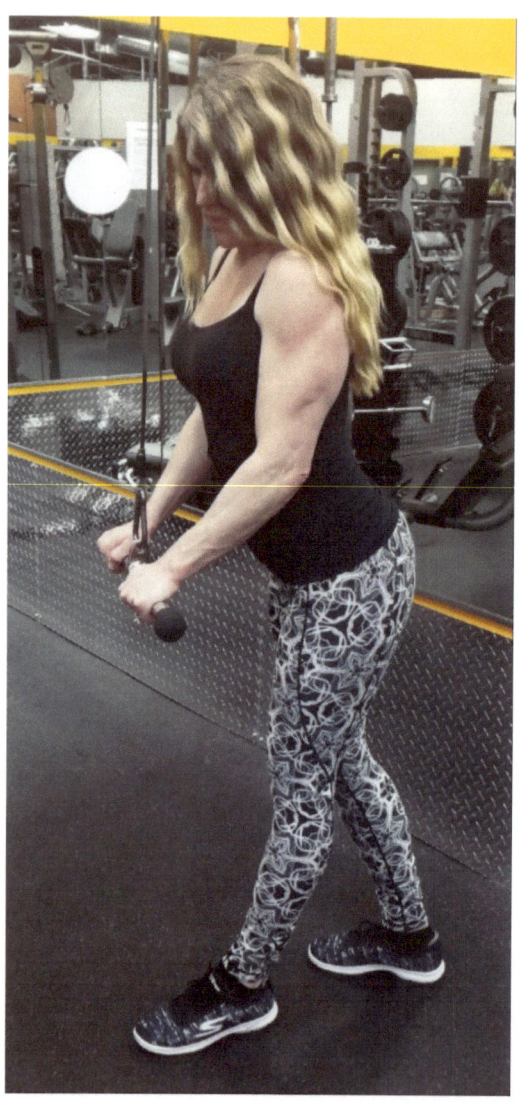

¾ of the way down still exhaling (blowing out) as you're pressing downward.

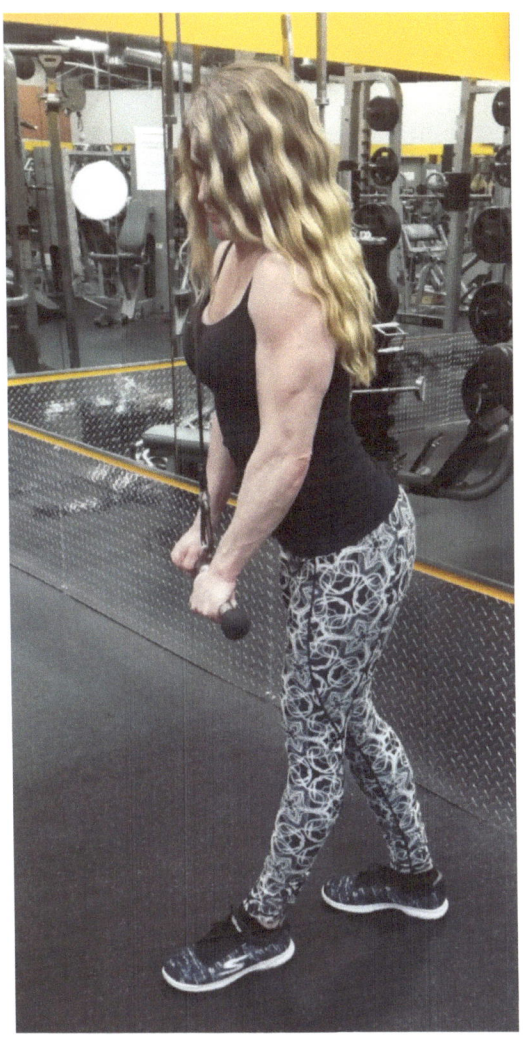

Fully exhale at the bottom and begin inhaling as you're returning to the original start position and repeat.

Dumbbell Hammer Curls

Now let's return for one more set of biceps and let's do a set of dumbbell hammer curls standing or sitting the choice is yours, and let's do another 4 sets of 25 reps for a total of 100 repetitions. Again only take a 60 second rest between sets unless you are training with a workout partner. Then only rest while they perform their set of 25 reps. Make each set of 25 repetitions a challenge.

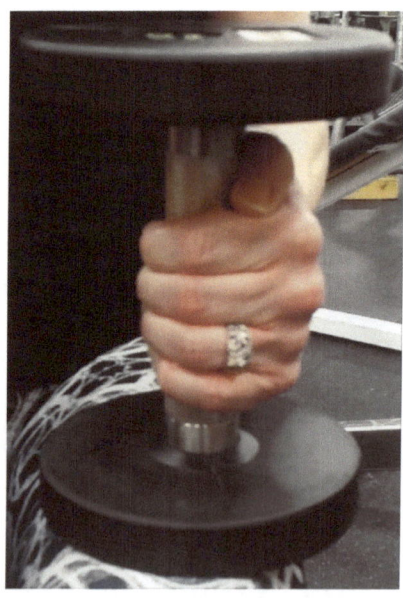

Hammer Curls Hand Position

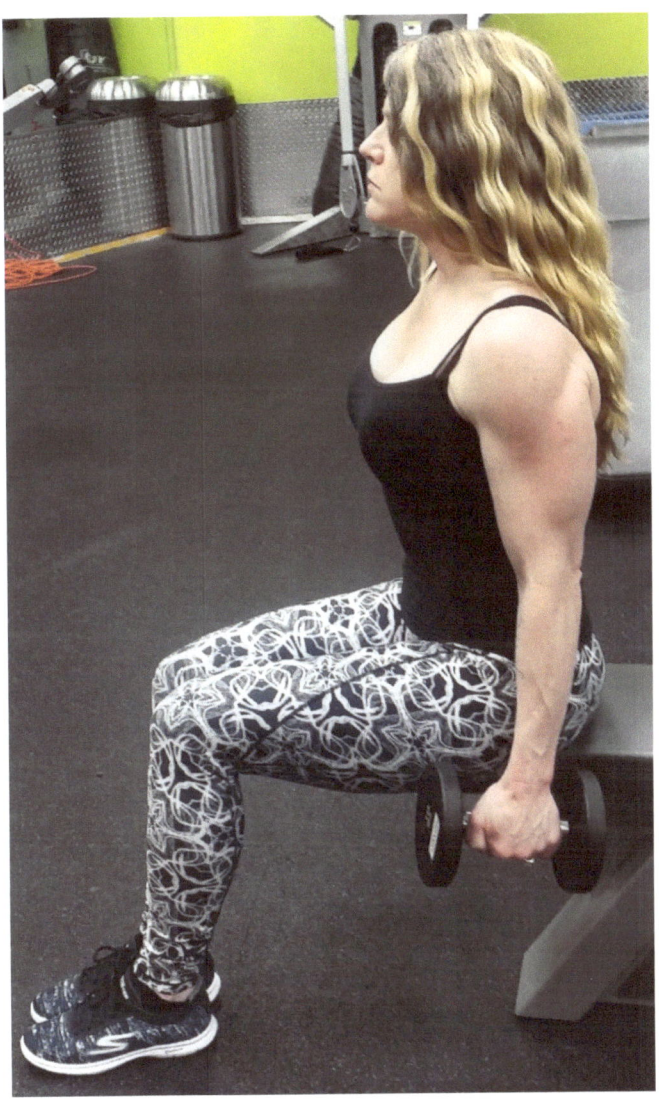

Take a deep breath and just before curling upward begin to slowly blow out.

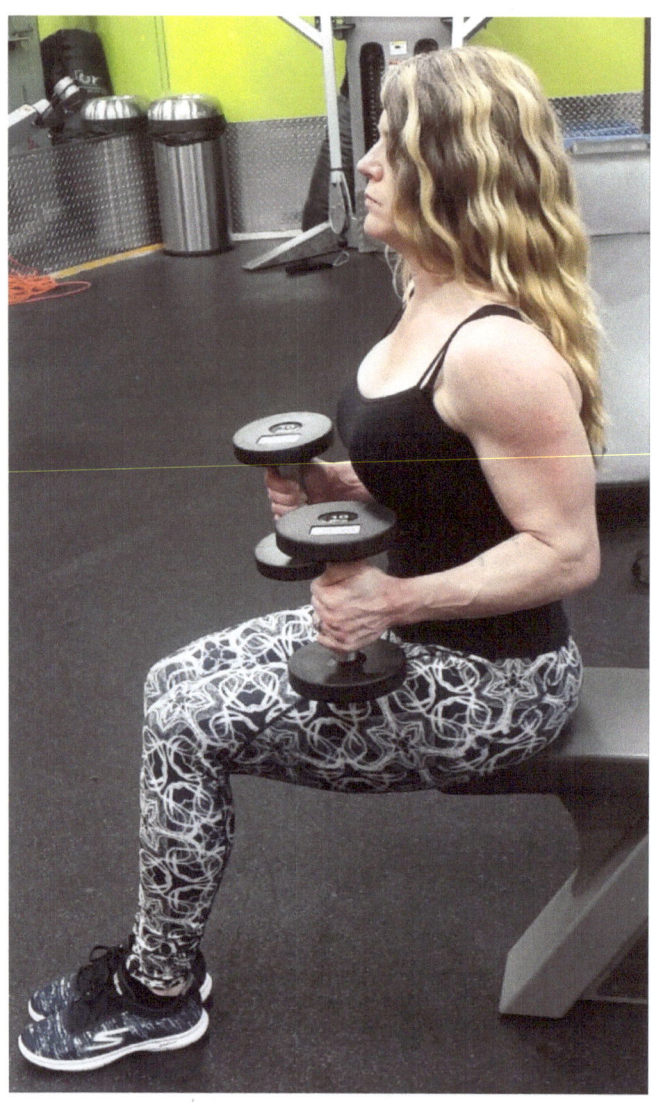

Continue blowing outward as you're curling the weight upward.

Women's Training Guide To Sexy Fit Arms
By Daryl BIG"D" Jones

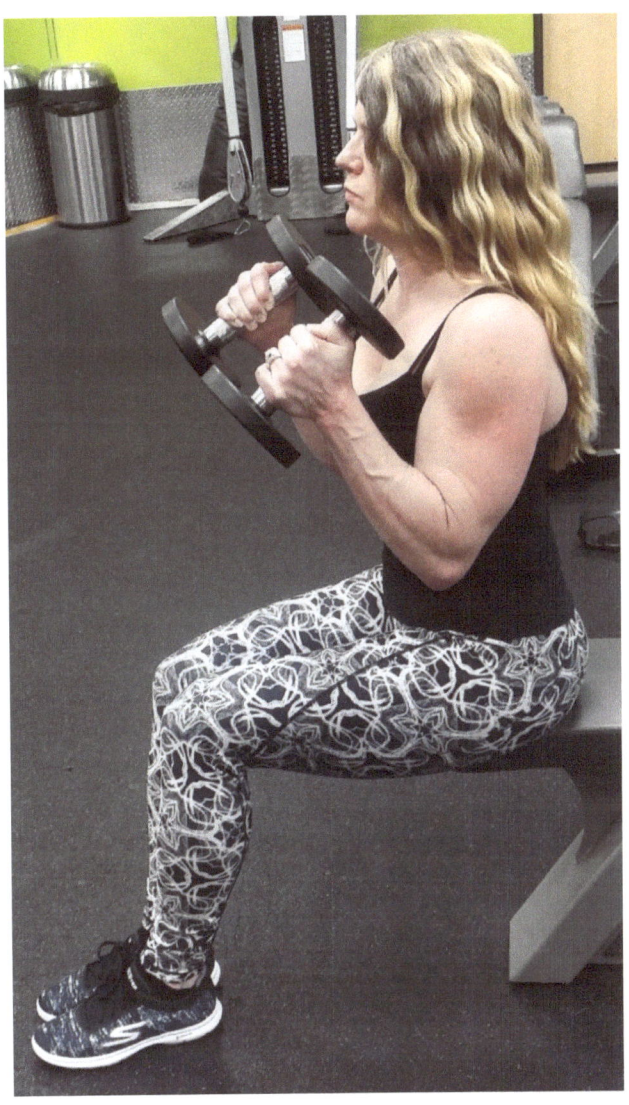

Fully exhale at the top of the movement and repeat. Do 4 sets of 25 reps for a total of 100 reps.

Body Weight Dips

Now for the final exercise of the day, we will move to body weight dips, here we will also do another 4 sets of 25 reps for a total of 100 repetitions. Make sure that at the bottom of each repetition we are going deep enough to really stress the triceps (backside of the upper arm) for change.

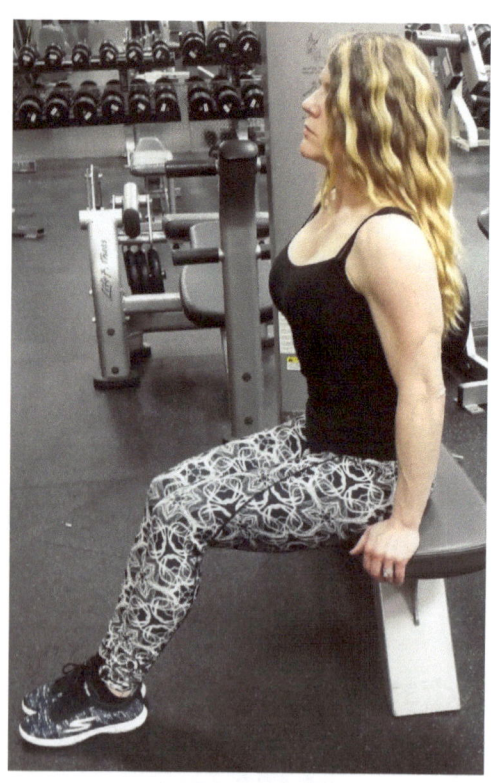

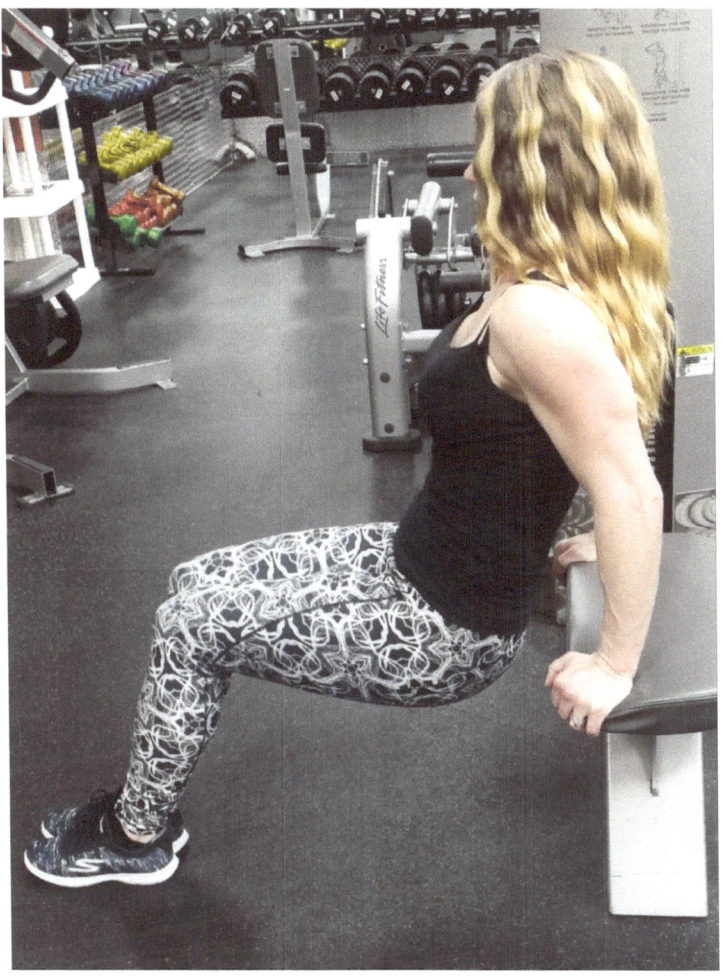

At the start position (shown above) begin to inhale as you are lowering yourself downward.

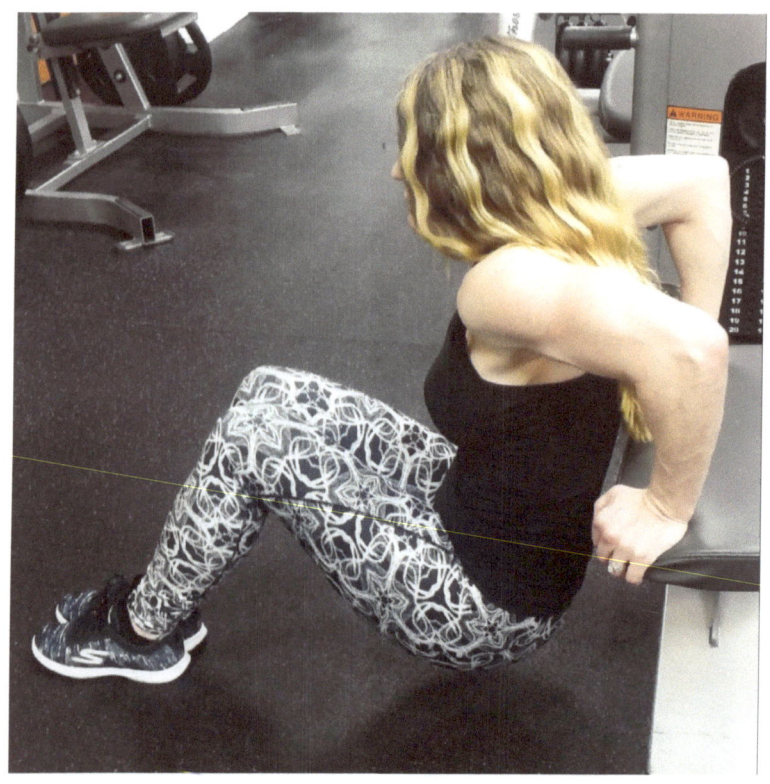

**Continue to inhale as you are lowering
your body downward.**

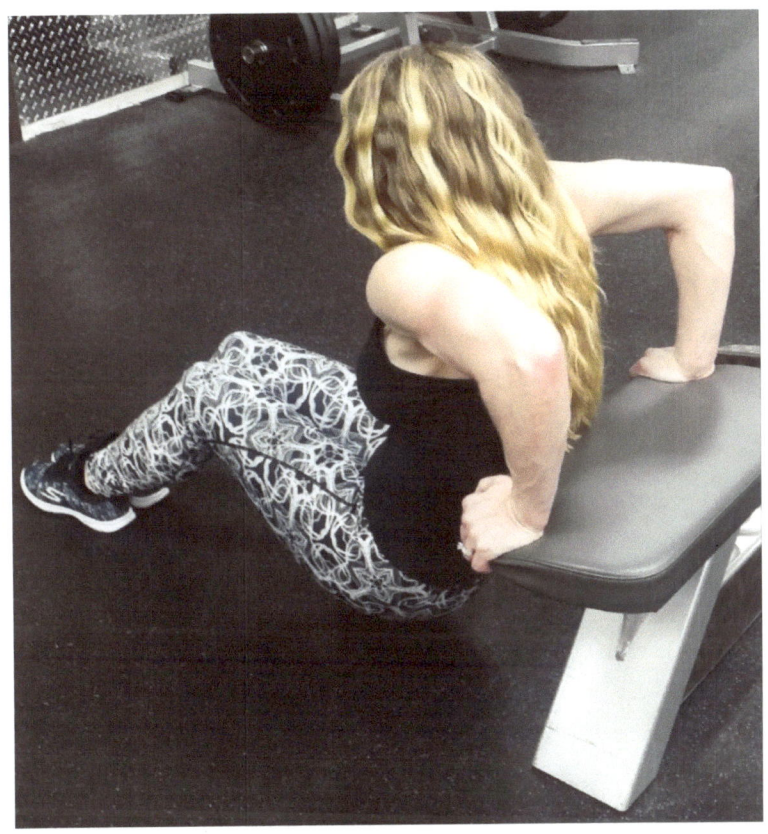

Now begin to blow out (exhale) as you are now beginning to press your body upward. Notice how the shoulder has dropped slightly below the elbow.

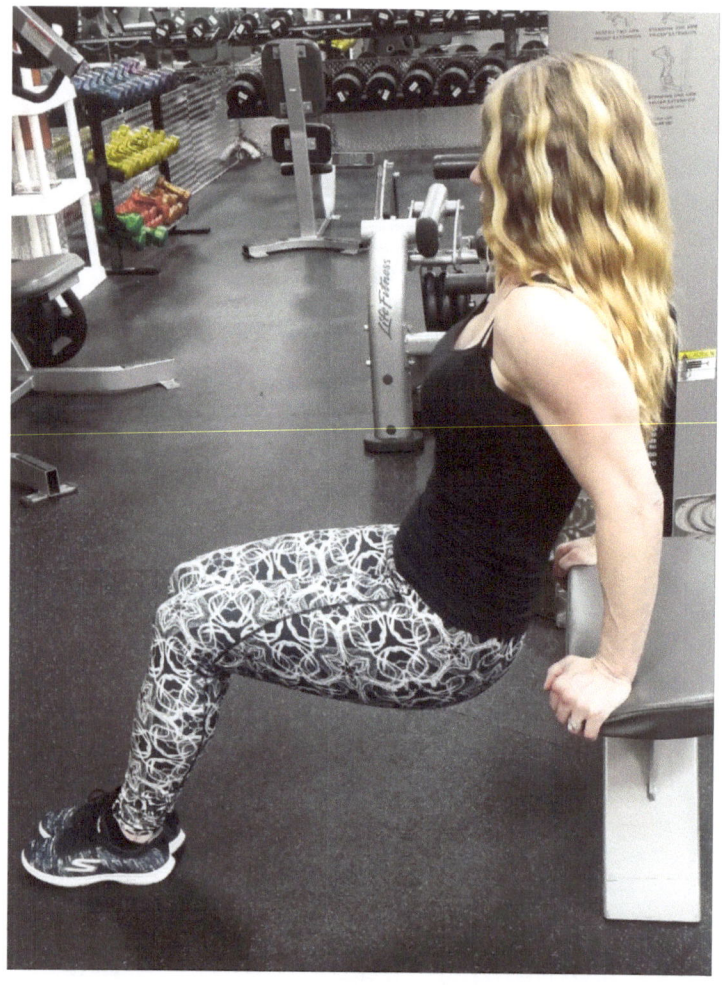

Fully exhale at the "top" of the movement and begin inhaling just before beginning the downward movement again.

Women's Training Guide To Sexy Fit Arms
By Daryl BIG"D" Jones

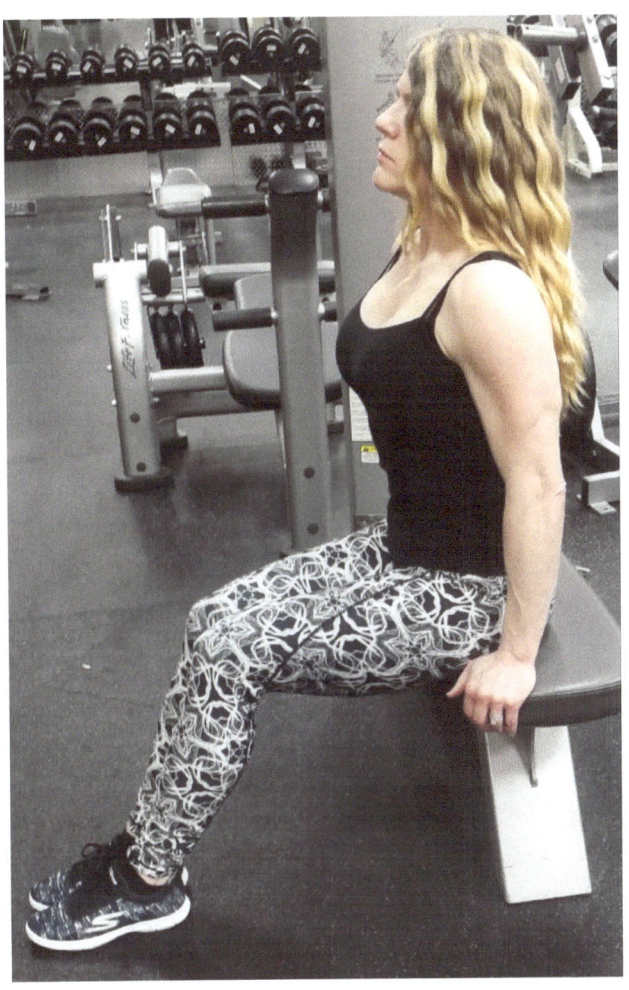

Do 4 sets of 25 repetitions for a total of 100 repetitions. Make sure to rest for "only" 60 seconds in between each set.

Women's Training Guide To Sexy Fit Arms
By Daryl BIG"D" Jones

Side Laterals

We will now do side laterals as the final exercise towards developing sexy fit arms. Side laterals are a shoulder (Side Deltoid) exercise that will change the look of any arm when performed correctly on a regular basis. This is an exercise that will separate the shoulders and arms with a nice athletic detailed cut. This exercise alone will help get rid of what I call a "SHARM" you may be asking yourself what the heck is a "SHARM" it's when a person has a shoulder and arm smoothly blended together into one long looking muscle. This lack of definition alone will destroy the potential look of an awesome set of arms. This separation looks great on a woman and will simply enhance the overall appearance of a nice set of "sexy" arms. So as all the above exercises we will be doing 4 sets of 25 repetitions for a total of 100 repetitions. Make sure to do your best and only rest for no longer than 60 seconds in between each set. Ladies you "can" do this. NOTE: You can do this without any weights until you get stronger for additional resistance.

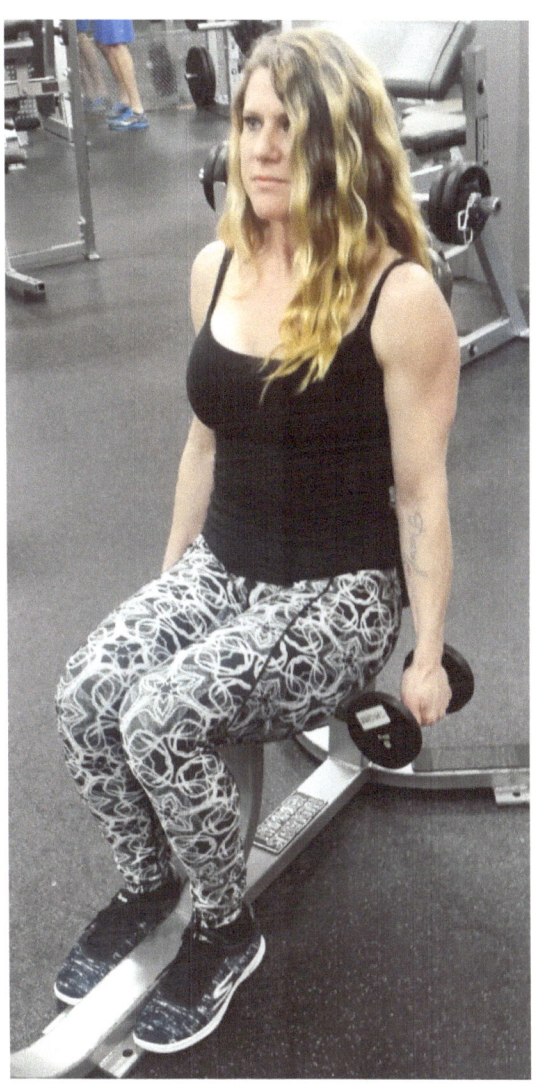

**Starting position, take a deep breath
before beginning the upward movement.**

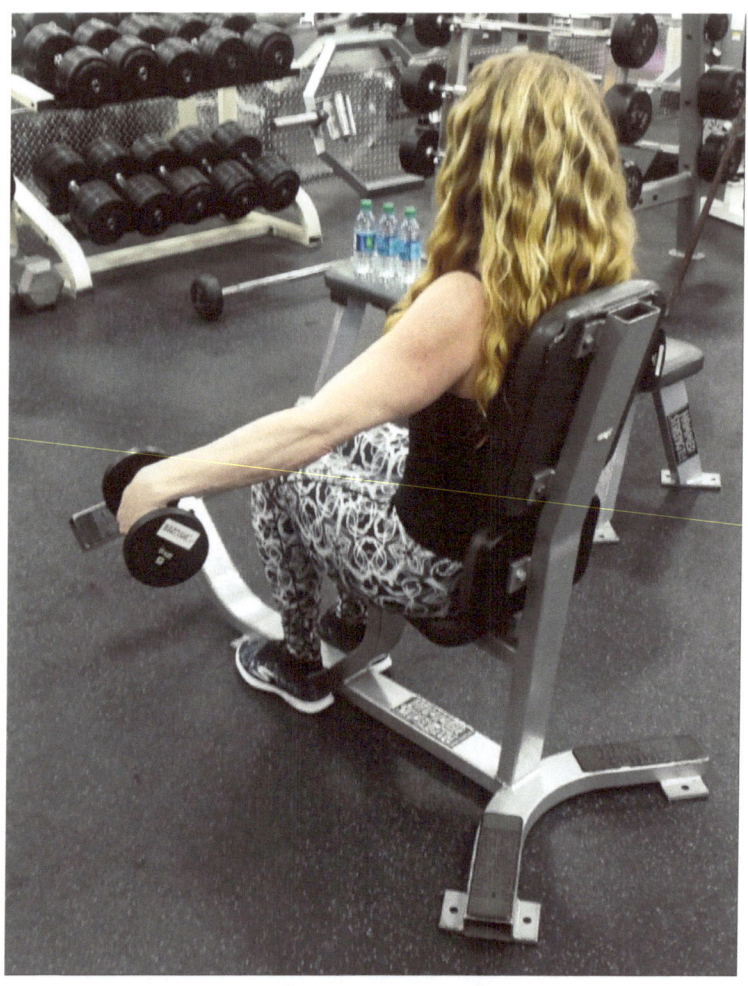

Exhale as you begin to lift upward. Lift up with a "wide" outward left to right reach, keeping the arms straight but without locking the joints. Keep a slight bend in the elbow.

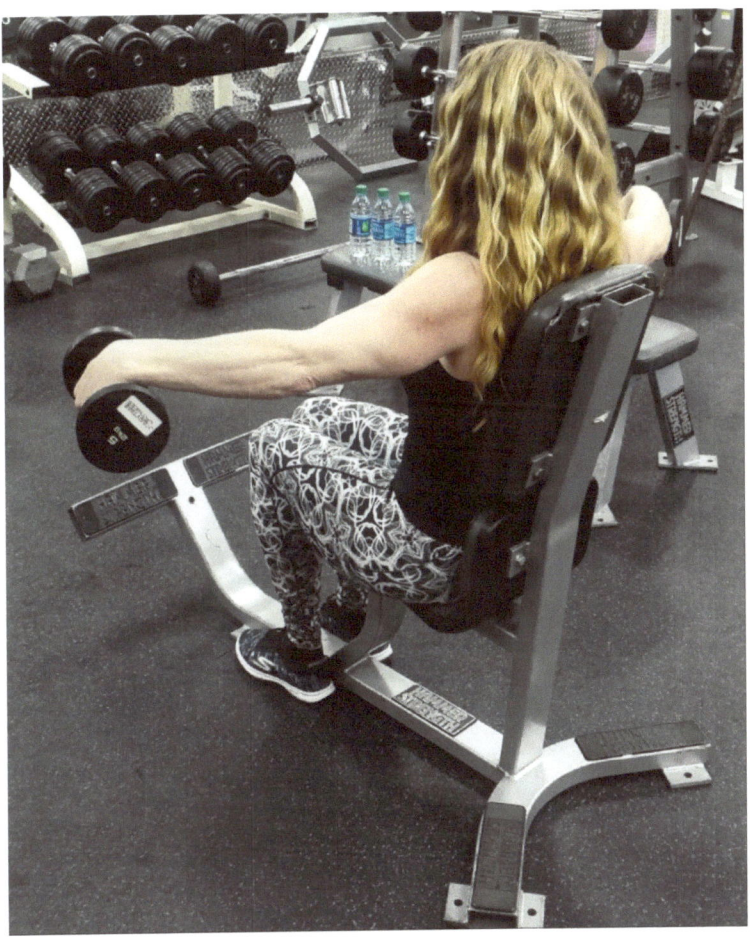

Continue to exhale as you are bringing the weights upward. Notice how the hands and wrist are bent downward, gripping the dumbbells in a hooking fashion.

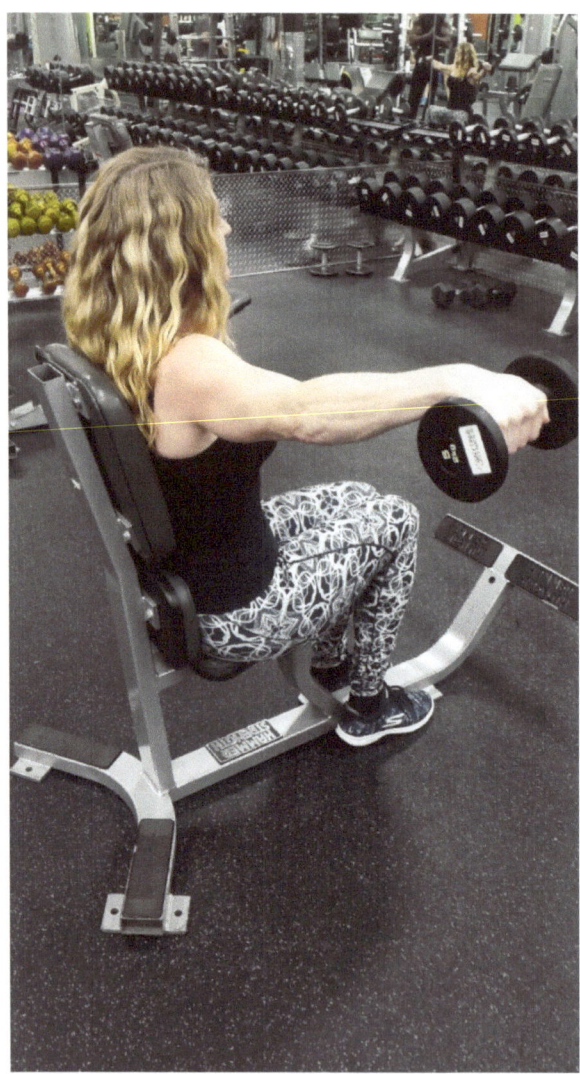

Here as we are now at the top of the movement, you'll notice how the elbow has come up equally as high as the shoulder.

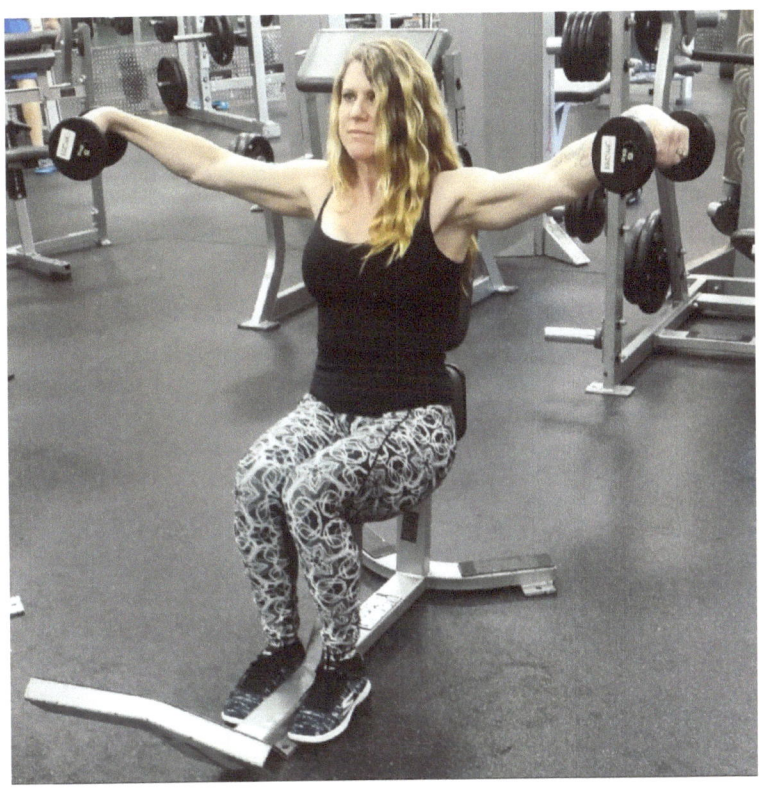

Fully exhale at the top of this movement and as you are now about to lower the arms in a controlled fashion, begin to inhale as the weight is being lowered. Again notice the bend in the wrist and the level of the elbow raising upward as high the shoulders themselves.

OBSTICLES

Success isn't measured by how many times you get knocked down, but rather how many times you get back up. Expect things to not go perfectly and don't get depressed or lose motivation simply because something unexpected happens. Always focus on the positive and don't brood on the negatives. You can overcome obstacles with some of these ideas:

If you miss a training day, simply start where you left off the very next day.

If you miss a scheduled meal don't eat two meals on the next scheduled eating time simply eat the next meal and go on from there.

If your time is limited beyond your normal control, don't miss the entire.

Women's Training Guide To Sexy Fit Arms
By Daryl BIG"D" Jones

Workout, simply go into the gym and train with the available time you have (don't miss the entire training if possible).

These simple approaches that should aide you in successfully achieving your fitness goals, just know none of us are perfect but try to always give 110% effort toward your goals and I'm absolutely sure you'll be happy with your final results.

Train Hard and Then Train Harder!

You now have all the tools you need to grow your own set of head-turning arms also known as guns. So now it's time to get in the gym and train hard – and after that, as I always say, then train even harder!

www.ingramcontent.com/pod-product-compliance
Lightning Source LLC
Chambersburg PA
CBHW050831290526
45792CB00001B/349